I0415606

Make Shampoos At Home Using Natural Ingredients

"Discover recipes for quality natural hair shampoos"

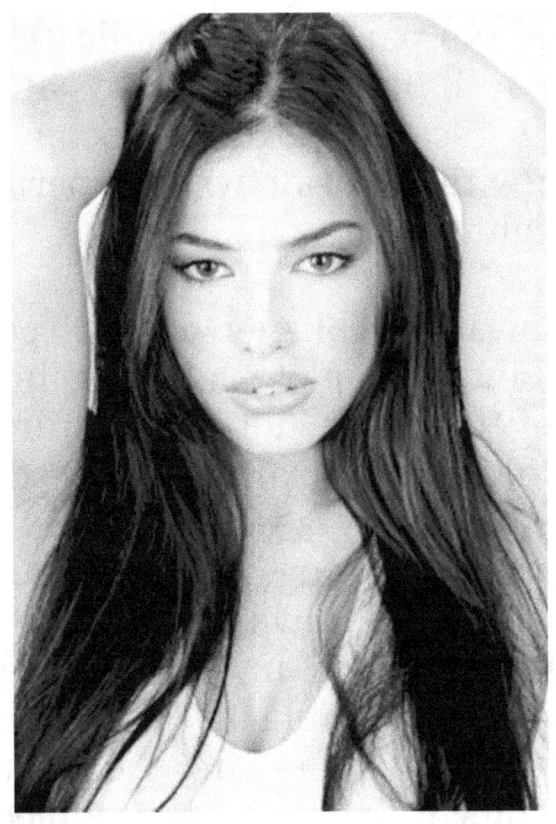

Rudy S Silva, Natural Nutritionist

Make Shampoos At Home Using Natural Ingredients © 2013 by Rudy S Silva

ISBN-13: 978-1492969709

ISBN-10: 1492969702

persons, people, or organizations are unintentional. In practical advice books, like anything else in life, there are no guarantees of income made.

All readers are advised to seek their own medical help.

The information here is for educational purposes and in no way is it medical advice or treatment. Ask your doctor before using any of the natural remedies listed here.

First Printing, 2012 Printed in the United States of America

Table of Contents

1: Why Make Your Own Shampoos?

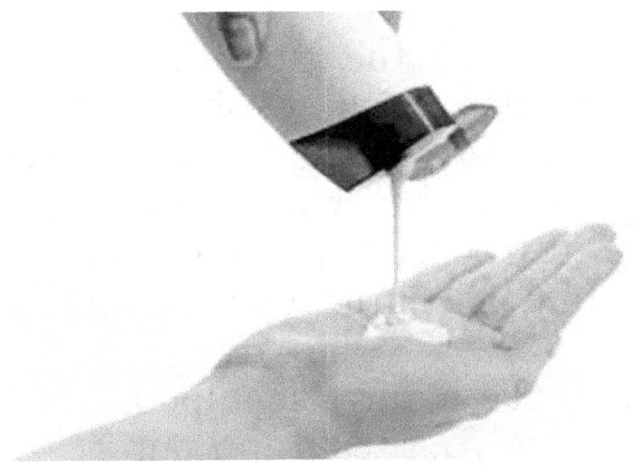

Many people are fed up with commercial shampoos. They want more natural shampoos that don't damage their hair or compromise their health. Commercial manufacturers don't want to do this, since they are making a good profit producing shampoos that harm you.

Using commercial shampoos all the time causes your hair to lose its minerals, such as calcium, phosphorous, iron and nitrogen. This is caused by the harsh chemicals these shampoos have. With chemicals clogging your scalp follicles and irritating your skin, this could eventually lead to hair thinning or permanent hair loss.

Keep in mind that the most important thing about shampoos is they should not have chemicals, which harm you. Having a shampoo that has the right pH is not any good, if it has petrochemicals and other harsh chemicals that will harm your hair and health.

When you make natural shampoos, they have the right pH for your scalp and skin.

You need to shampoo your hair every day with a good shampoo. Dirt, grime, and oil accumulate on your scalp and hair each day. Your scalp is constantly producing new skin cells and shedding old cells to its surface. Shampooing removes daily grime accumulation and this allows your hair to breathe and grow properly.

Now, there are many so-called natural shampoos that are much better and do contain less of what will harm you. The problem is that they are more expense that commercial shampoos.

However, now you can make your own shampoos the way you want with the herbs and natural products that you chose. You won't be using any fake or un-natural fragrances, dyes, or preservatives.

Naturopathic doctors always tell you that whatever you put on your skin will end up in your blood. You shouldn't put anything on your skin that you cannot eat. All the products that you use in this book, you can drink except for the natural soap solution.

Commercial shampoos contain all kinds of chemicals that are designed to make the shampoo look, smell, and flow smoothly. When you buy a shampoo, you want it to flow out of the bottle easily, smell pretty, and to lather up quickly and fully.

You want a shampoo that cleans your hair no matter what condition your hair is in. To do all the things you want requires shampoo manufacturers to put all kinds of chemicals and additives into their shampoo. These chemicals will eventually cause thinning hair, excess hair loss, and contribute to poor health.

Hair Vitamins

Most commercial shampoos don't have a lot of minerals or vitamins. When you make your own shampoos, the herbs you use will contain many minerals, vitamins, anti-oxidants, and hundreds of other phytonutrients. So how can you get these nutrients into your scalp? Some of them will penetrate your skin and feed your scalp cells and hair naturally. But, other nutrients will not penetrate your scalp.

For the nutrients that are not absorbed into your scalp naturally, you will find in the following chapter one nutrient that will act as a transporter to help you move more nutrients into your scalp.

Here is a list of some of the important nutrients your hair needs to have good health. These nutrients not only keep your hair healthy, but help you minimize hair loss. You can also supplement with these vitamins to give your hair a boost from the blood flow to your scalp.

Vitamin A

Vitamin A (Retinol) – herbs that you will be using have this vitamin. You can take between 10,000 – 25,000 IU's

B Vitamins

Many herbs contain some of the B vitamins. The B vitamins are essential for minimizing hair loss. When you supplement with these vitamins, it is best to use a complete B vitamin supplement such as the B100's. Remember, you need B vitamins every day. Your body will only use the Bs it needs and excrete the excess. This is why your urine will be a deep yellow, since the excess Bs are being eliminated. These are the most important B vitamins for your hair.

Vitamin B1 (Thiamin)

Vitamin B12 (Cobalt)
Vitamin B2 (Riboflavin)
Vitamin B5 (Pantothenic Acid)
Vitamin B6 (Pyridoxine)
Vitamin B9 (Folic Acid)

Vitamin H (Biotin) – this is a B vitamin and is a very important hair-loss vitamin. It is found in some herbs. Lack of this vitamin shows up as thinning hair and loss of hair. So, you should make sure you are supplementing with it, if you want to have good hair health.

However, Biotin should be used and taken with the other B vitamins to get the best absorption. Use around 300 mcg and if the B100 do not have enough biotin, you may have to supplement with biotin separately.

Vitamin C

Some herbs will have vitamin C. A good amount vitamin C to take every day is around 3000 to 4000 mg. You can always tell when you are taking too much vitamin C, since your stools will get softer or watery. Use the buffered type or Ester C to avoid stomach aches. This will cost you quite a bit more.

Vitamin E

You can add vitamin E to your shampoos by breaking a few capsules open and putting them into your shampoo. Use 400 – 800 IU of vitamin E, but do not exceed the 800mg. Use the Alpha tocopherols, since they are the most active form of this vitamin. You will see this form listed as alpha-tocopheryl acetate.

2: Detrimental Ingredients In Drugstore Shampoos

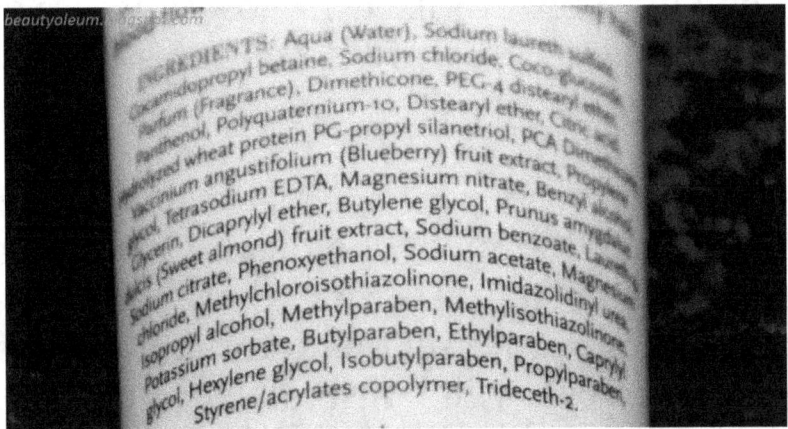

If you are still using commercial shampoos, take a look at the shampoo you are using and see if any of following ingredients shows up. If you are using a more natural shampoo, these ingredients may not show up.

You will find that commercial shampoos have a long list of ingredients. You may not know what these ingredients are or do and may not even be able to pronounce them. If you use a more natural shampoo, their ingredient list will be shorter.

Here is a list of some of the ingredients you will find in your typical shampoos, creams, sprays, lotions or cosmetics. There are hundreds if not thousands of these types of ingredients that are used in cosmetics. Some of these ingredients are sometimes found in food.

This list gives you some idea as to how harmful commercial shampoo chemicals are to your health. The harm, from these chemicals, comes when you use them for a long time. These chemicals will cause disease, and when they do, you will not know that the disease came from using these chemicals.

Acrylates – (Acrylate, Acrylamide, Butylaminoethyl, Methylacrylate polymer) - these polymers are synthetic and are used many creams, shampoos, and nail lacquers. Animal testing has shown that these polymers are linked to tumors and can cause various skin and allergic reactions.

Ammonium Lauryl Sulfate – this is a petrochemical combined with an ammonium compound – one of the least desirable synthetic detergents.

Benzoic Acid, Sodium Benzoate – benzoic is used in cosmetics and foods as a preservative. This chemical, in low amounts, has been related to brain damage, neurological disorders, and cancer.

BHA and BHT – Butylated hydroxyanisole and butylated hydroxytoluene are synthetic antioxidants used in cosmetics. These chemicals contain the toxin toluene and should be avoided.

Cocamide DEA, Cocamidopropyl Betaine – these are synthetic detergents.

Cocamidopropylamine Oxide – this chemical is added to shampoos to lower their pH.

Disodium EDTA – FDA does not consider this chemical to be harmful and it is not readily absorbed by the skin. However, when combined with other chemicals it enhances their skin absorption characteristics.

Hydrolyzed Animal Elastin, Hydrolyzed Animal Protein Sorbitol - the hydrolyzed animal extracts contain proteins to repair your hair. But, this formula contains too many synthetic chemicals for it to be of any value for your hair.

Imiazolidinyl Urea – there is some concern that this chemical is toxic and carcinogenic, since it's a proven formaldehyde releaser. The Cosmetic Ingredient Review (CIR) Expert Panel after their investigation, considers this chemical safe at a maximum concentration of .5%.

Lauramide DEA – these are chemicals that come from petrochemicals and are harmful to your hair and health.

Methylchloroisothiazolinone – this is a chemical that many people are allergic to. If you have sensitive skin make sure your shampoo does not have it.

Methylisothiazolinone – this product was tested on rats and rabbits and they found that it was safe when used in "rinse-off" products, provided they do not exceed 15 ppm.

Methylparaben – is considered a moderate concern, since it creates endocrine disruptions and cellular changes. It can mimic estrogen and can act as a hormone.

Mineral Oil, Paraffin, and Petrolatum - come from petroleum products. They are toxic, clog pores, and lead to skin problems. They disrupt skin growth and may cause cancer.

Parabens, Propylparaben – are para-hydroxybenzoic acid esters (methyl, propyl, butyl) – these chemicals are toxic and are connected with the cause of cancer. They also disrupt hormone activity by mimicking estrogen.

Phenol, Phenoxyethanol Phenolcarbolic acid – Phenolic compounds are used as a preservative in lotions and skin creams. They are toxic and can cause paralysis, convulsions, and coma when inhaled in large quantities.

Polyquaternium 10 – has low toxicity and has been found to irritate the eyes.

Propylene Glycol – propylene glycol is a synthetic chemical and comes from petroleum. In cosmetics, it attracts water so it is used as a surfactant, solvent, moisturizer, humectant, and as a carrier in fragrance oils.

It is also used in as brake fluid and antifreeze. It is toxic and causes allergic reactions, skin irritations, and affects the health of the liver and kidney.

Quaternium-15, – this is formaldehyde, which is carcinogenic in high amounts and can be an irritant to your skin, eyes and respiratory system.

Quaternium-22 – has been identified as contaminated with impurities, which are linked to cancer and other health issues.

Silk Amino Acids (Hydrolyzed Silk Protein) – provide amino acids to your scalp and hair and are not considered toxic to your body.

Sodium C14-16 Olefin Sulfonate – is a detergent that may cause eye, skin, and respiratory system irritation.

Sodium laurel, lauryl sulfate, SLS, sodium laureth sulfate, SLES – is a chemical used in thousands of cosmetic products – shampoos, lotions, creams. It is a strong degreaser, which dries your hair and skin and can cause hair loss. It is also found in many cleaning products.

Soyatrimonium Chloride – considered an irritant for the skin, eyes, and lungs.

3: How To Make Natural Shampoos

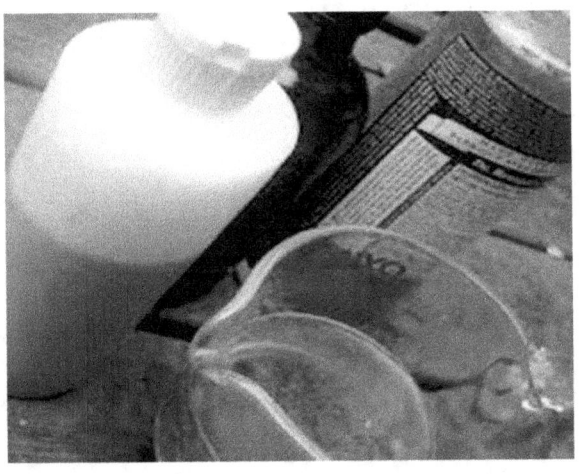

Here is how to make your shampoos. In this chapter, you will find out how to make the base shampoo. You will then use this base shampoo to make other shampoos that are specific to what you are trying to accomplish with your hair. The base shampoo is strong enough to clean both your scalp and hair. Normally, you need a shampoo for your scalp and one for your hair. In the following chapters, you will find out how to make a shampoo for your scalp, when you have scalp or dandruff problems.

The base shampoo is composed of the following ingredients:

8 oz. plastic clear bottle
Castile liquid soap
MSM torpedoes
Apple cider vinegar
Rosemary herb for dark hair, Chamomile for light hair
Sweet basil herb,
Ginger root

8 oz. Plastic Clear Bottle

Try to use a clear plastic bottle. You can also use a glass bottle, if you like. You may be using small amounts of oils, so you want a bottle that can tolerate oils. Some plastic bottles are not for use with oils. You can buy them at a health-food store. Try not to use a "used bottle" that had other cosmetics in it. You want to have a clean bottle to make sure you don't have bacterial, fungal, or other contaminates in the bottle.

Castile Liquid Soap

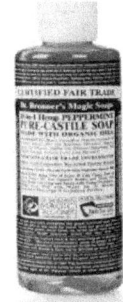

Castile liquid soap is the center of this natural shampoo. It has a lot of different uses other than for shampoos, since it is a soap base. Castile soap comes from olive oil and has been around for hundreds of years. You can buy Castile soap with plain, peppermint, eucalyptus, almond, rose, citrus, lavender, and tea tree scents. It comes in a variety of sizes, but I recommend you start with a **32 oz. bottle of castile** soap.

MSM torpedoes

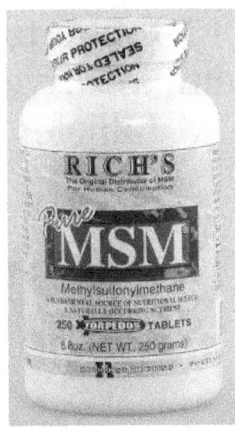

MSM is a sulfur compound called MethylSulfynolMethane or MSM. This nutrient is used by every body cell and is considered an anti-aging supplement because it will keep you young inside and out.

When MSM is embedded in your cell membranes, it keeps your cells flexible and prevents them from becoming hard and dry.

This allows nutrients to go into the cells and wastes and toxins to come out easily.

Wastes that do not totally come out of your cells cause inflammation and disease. You should also add this nutrient to your daily supplement use.

In your scalp, MSM Increases blood circulation, has Anti-inflammatory action, and helps Soften collagen.

MSM provides organic sulfur to your scalp, which improves the health and strength of your hair. But, most importantly, **MSM acts as a transport** and deliver system to drive herbal nutrients into your scalp and follicles, where they can do the most good.

Here's where you can buy the **MSM torpedoes**, 1000 mg, 250 count.

Apple Cider Vinegar – Bragg

Here is another miracle product. This product has so many uses and benefits for your health.

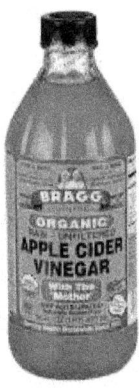

In shampoos, apple cider vinegar is used as a preservative, as a guard against bacterial growth, and as a provider of amazing nutrients.

This natural vinegar is filled with minerals and various nutrients. Your follicles and hair are always in need of minerals. When your body needs minerals, and you don't have a good store of these in your body, your hair will not get the minerals it needs. Your hair is the last place where your body sends nutrients. Eat a good diet to prevent hair loss.

Here are some of the nutrients in apple cider vinegar.

- thirteen types of carbolic acids

- four aldehydes

- twenty ketones

- eighteen types of alcohols

- eight ethyl acetates

It has acetic acid, propionic acid, lactic acid, enzymes, amino acids as well as roughage in the form of potash and apple pectin.

It has these minerals, trace elements and vitamins.

Potassium, Calcium, Magnesium, Phosphorous, Chlorine, Sodium, Sulfur, Copper, Iron, Silicon, Fluorine Vitamin C, Vitamin E, Vitamin A, Vitamin B1, Vitamin B2, Vitamin B6, Provitamin beta-carotene, Vitamin P.

Rosemary Herb

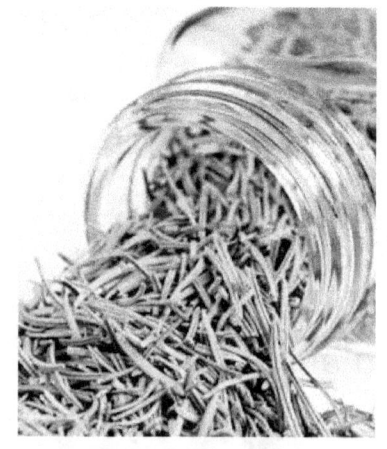 Here is an herb worthy of being in the base solution you will use for your targeted shampoos. The rosemary herb leaves stimulate the hair follicles and help keep them healthy. It strengthens your hair and its nutritional value is outstanding. It contains

vitamins A and C, B-6, riboflavin, thiamin, folate, niacin, and pantothenic acid.

Rosemary also contains fatty acids and phytoesterols, and 18 amino acids, the building blocks of protein, which are excellent for your hair.

It contains Calcium, iron, phosphorous, manganese, magnesium, potassium, sodium, zinc and copper in small amounts.

Buy one oz of rosemary herb. This should be enough to a few bottles of shampoo.

Basil Leaves Herb

Basil is antibacterial and is good for insect bites, parasites, and worms. It is used for skin or scalp sores.

Ginger root

Ginger root is great for blood circulation. Adding it to the base shampoo will help give you little blood

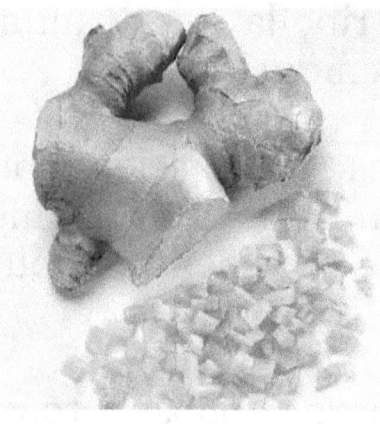

circulation around your hair follicles. It also is good for dandruff and for an itchy scalp.

Ginger is also a great source of nutrients. It contains small traces of B vitamins, vitamin C, E, and K. It also has an array of different fats and fatty acids. It has small traces of 10 different minerals and 18 amino acids. All of these nutrients are great for hair health.

Making The Base Shampoo

Here is the step by step process for making the base shampoo.

1. Mix one heaping tablespoon of each rosemary and basil herbs in a mason jar, which has a lid.

2. Boil 1 1/2 cups of distilled water and add 4 to 5 slices of ginger that is peeled. Also add 2 tablespoons of the mixed herbs into

the boiling water. Let the ginger and herbs simmer for 10 minutes with the cover slightly ajar, then let this solution sit for another 10 to 15 minutes. You want to have some of the water boil off, so that your herbal mixture will be more concentrated.

3. After 20 minutes or so and the herb mixture has cooled a little, strain the herbal mixture into a bowl or a pouring glass. The remaining liquid should be around 4 to 8 oz.

4. Now, put 2000 to 3000 mg of MSM into the herb mixture. After the MSM has dissolved, the mixture is ready to go into a 8 or 16 oz. bottle. Do not put MSM into boiling water, since the Sulfur in the MSM is quite volatile.

5. With the herbal mixture and MSM cooled and ready to pour into the bottle, add 2 to 3 tablespoons of apple cider vinegar into

the bottle.

6. Pour 4 oz. of herbal tea into the 8 oz plastic bottle. If you are using a 16 oz. bottle, pour 8 oz. of herb tea into that bottle. Use from 1/3 to 1/2 herbal tea in your bottle. The rest will be Castile.

7. Now, pour Castile liquid soap to almost fill the bottle. Cap the bottle and shake to mix the ingredients. Now you can label the bottle with the type of shampoo you have made. Make sure you pour the Castile soap last into the bottle to avoid creating a lot of bubbles in the bottle.

The shampoo is now finished and ready for use. Use this as a base for all of the shampoos you make. You can add different herbs to this shampoo to make different shampoos designed to deal with your different hair issues. In the following chapters, you will see how to make other shampoos.

pH Of Shampoo

The ideal pH of a shampoo is a neutral or slightly acidic. This is the pH you need for normal or oily hair. When you test your shampoo with litmus paper and find it is 7.0 it is neutral. If it is 6.70 to 6.99 pH, it is slightly acidic. An acidic shampoo is good for dry and damaged hair. This shampoo can shrink the cuticle and can make the hair stronger and shinier. The cuticle is a scale like cell that cover the hair shaft.

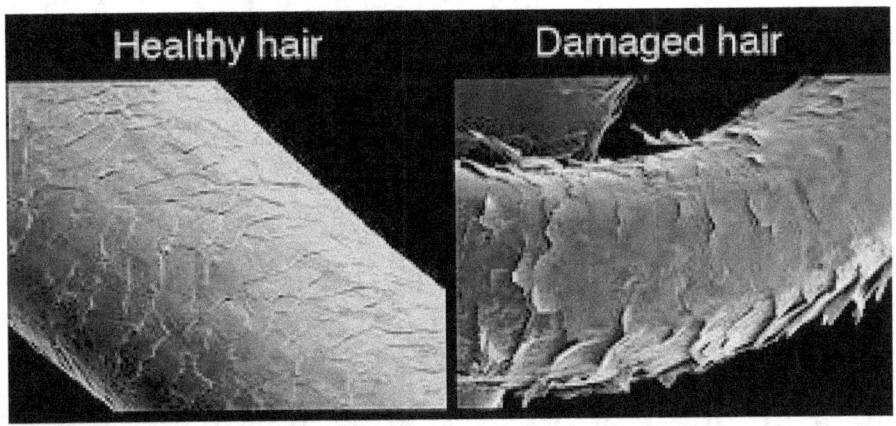

Many commercial shampoos are not pH balanced to neutral but are alkaline – a pH that is above 7.0. In this case, this shampoo makes your hair shaft swollen, weak, and flaky. It can make your hair look dull and feel lifeless. For this kind of hair you need a shampoo that is more acidic or with a pH of 6.50 and not 7.10 to 7.50. Here is a good **litmus pH paper** to use. It has pH steps of .25 and it will help you identify your shampoo's pH. The shampoos you make here are all slightly acidic.

Herbs In The Following Chapter

In the following chapters, you will find many different herbs listed and what they do for your scalp or hair. From this list, you can target the type of shampoo you want to create.

One thing to keep in mind is the color of your hair. If you have light colored hair, then some herbs may darken your hair. With any shampoo that you make, always do a hair test on a small portion of your hair to see if the shampoo will change the color of your hair.

4: Shampoos For Your Scalp

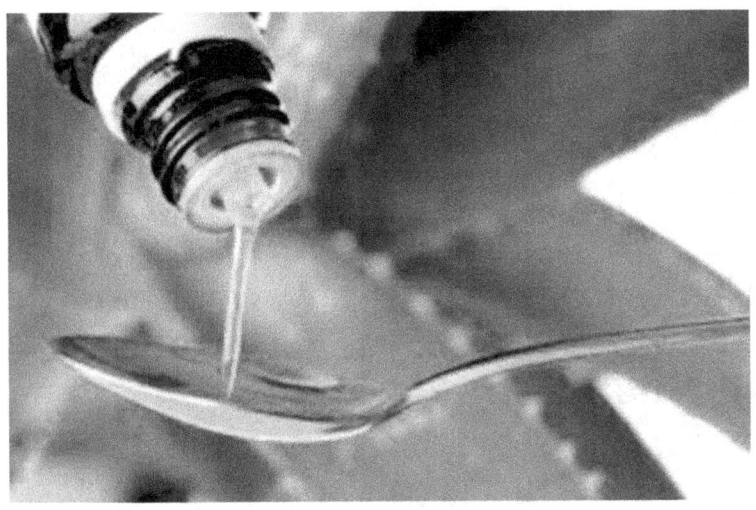

You will be making two shampoos, one for your scalp and one for your hair. The shampoo for your scalp is for various conditions that you might have with your scalp that you want to correct. If you don't have any scalp conditions that need help, then just the basic scalp shampoo is what you need. This basic shampoo will be one that can provide you with nutrients that will improve your hair and scalp health.

To make a powerful scalp shampoo, you want to add three or four more herbs to the base shampoo that can help make your scalp healthier.

Here are some recipes for scalp shampoos:

First make the Basic Scalp Shampoo as outlined in chapter 3. However, when you come to steps 1 and 3, you will be adding the new herbs to make different scalp shampoos.

Basic Shampoo

- 8 oz. plastic clear bottle
- Castile liquid soap
- MSM torpedoes
- Apple cider vinegar
- Rosemary herb
- Sweet basil herb
- Ginger root

Standard Scalp Recipe

Add any of these two herbs to your base shampoo to make a better scalp shampoo. Check what each herbs does and choose the one that makes sense to you.

Burdock Root – provides scalp circulation

Chaparral – increases the circulation of your scalp.

Comfrey leaves – give relief to an irritated scalp.

Eucalyptus – heals scalp irritation. It can help in regulating sebum production and cleans scalp and pores. It is also an anti-inflammatory.

Hyssop - can be used for treating scalp irritations, burns, or psoriasis.

Lavender flowers – is a gentle herb that helps to keep the proper hair pH and promotes the body and shine of your hair. It controls the production of sebaceous gland oil and reduces itchy and flaky scalp conditions. It also adds a flowery scent.

Nettles or Stinging Nettles – cleans and stimulates the scalp.

Sage - is used as a skin purifier and toner in shampoos. It is for greasy skin and provides fragrance. It has microbial action.

Yarrow - has a soothing effect on the skin and is anti inflammatory and non phototoxic.

Oily Hair Shampoo

Oily hair results from an overactive scalp sebaceous gland. If you have oily hair, you may have to wash it twice a day. When you use these natural shampoos, it will not be a problem to wash that frequently.

To the base shampoo, add any of one of the following herbs. The base shampoo will work as a shampoo for oily hair, but you can add one to three of the following herbs to make it a stronger "For oily hair shampoo."

It is not recommend that you add any essential oils to this shampoo. However, it is possible that certain oils may help cure the excess production of sebum. This can only be determined by your experimentation with the oils listed in the following chapters.

Betulla – is used for greasy or oily hair. It has anti-inflammatory properties and is also used as a fragrance.

Lemon balm – helps to remove excess oil and sebum.

Lemongrass – helps to clean your scalp by removing excess oil and sebum.

Sage – will reduce the formation of sebum in the sebaceous glands and provides scalp circulation. It is also good for hair growth.

Yarrow – reduces the production of sebum in the sebaceous glands.

If you need more herb choices, check the following chapters for the list of herbs to use.

5: Shampoos For Your Hair

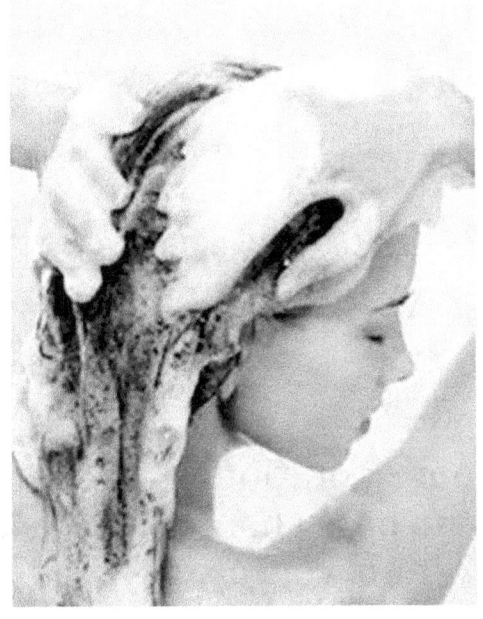

In this chapter, you will learn how to prepare shampoos for your hair. The base shampoo is an excellent shampoo for your hair. This shampoo and other shampoos you make here will be thinner than commercial shampoos. But these shampoos will clean your scalp and hair of excess oil and dirt, while conditioning your hair with herbs you use.

Here is the base shampoo formula

8 oz. plastic clear bottle

Castile liquid soap

MSM torpedoes

Apple cider vinegar

Rosemary herb

Sweet basil herb

Ginger root

Here are some additional herbs you can use and add to the base shampoo. Use these herbs for the condition you are trying to correct in your hair.

To add some fragrance to your shampoo, try the following herbs. Make an infusion of two to three of these herbs and simmer to concentrate the tea. Add these herbs to your shampoo.

Fragrance

Mints such as **peppermint** and **spearmint**

are used as fragrances. They are also a scalp stimulant and antiseptic.

Lemon grass - has been used as a fragrance, but also has minerals.

Lavender - can be used as fragrance. It controls the production of sebaceous gland oil and reduces itchy and flaky scalp conditions

Check the list of herbs to use for more fragrant herbs.

Hair strengthening and health

Use these herbs to improve the health of your hair.

Arnica – contain linolenic acid, vitamins A, B, C, and D. Used as a hair tonic and as a fragrance.

Coltsfoot contains silica and cysteine which is beneficial for hair health.

Hawthorn - is an astringent and can be used

as a hair tonic.

Kelp - contains a high level of mineral salts, vitamins and amino acids that are good for hair health.

Lemon grass - has been used as a fragrance, but also has minerals.

Horsetail – contains silica, which strengthens your hair shaft. It also stimulates blood circulation of your scalp.

Marshmallow root – provides hair with a conditioning effect.

Pre hair conditioner

If you want to strengthen your hair, you can use ginger root. Juice ginger root and massage it into your scalp. Let it sit on our scalp for 10 to 15 minutes. Then, you can shampoo your hair.

6: Natural Dandruff And Hair Loss Shampoos

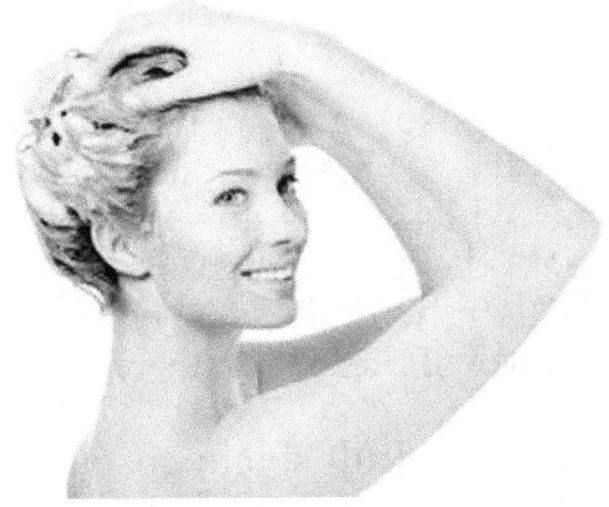

Commercial dandruff shampoos are considered the most dangerous shampoos that you can use. They contain toxic chemicals that prevent your scalp from peeling, such as selenium sulfide, cadmium sulfide, polythionates, hexachlorophene or bithionol. These chemical get into your blood, when you have it in your shampoo.

Some of these dandruff shampoo formulations

are only available through prescription, but some are on your drug store shelves. If you constantly use these shampoo, it will cause liver and organ damage.

Dandruff shampoos also contain the toxic chemicals creosol and polyvinyl pyrrlidone plastic, PVP. Some of them contain zinc pyrithione, which slows down cell growth and holds back the yeast organism that causes dandruff. Some contain salicylic acid, sulfur or a combination of these various chemicals.

Many of the dandruff shampoos are not made for light hair. If you have blonde, light brown, bleached or gray hair chances are dandruff shampoos will darken your hair. Always check the label on this type of shampoo to see what the limitations are.

Use herbs for your dandruff shampoo that have antifungal, anti-bacteria, and anti-parasitic properties. It has been found that many dandruff conditions are caused by a fungus infection. However, the poor diet and having poor scalp blood circulation prevents your hair from getting the nutrients it needs to keep healthy. So take the time to learn the basics of a good nutritional diet.

Dandruff Shampoo

Many people suffer from dandruff disease. When you have dandruff, the scalp skin forms a scale that does not easily rinse, powder or come off.

Normally dead skin is pushed up to the scalp surface where it eventually becomes a powder and dissolves in a shampoo or water and is rinsed away.

Whereas, the scales of dandruff do not form a powder and become harden. Their large formation makes them visible, and they flake off your hair and get on your clothes near your hair.

If you prepare a shampoo, and it does not solve your dandruff problem, formulate another shampoo. One formulation may not work for you, because of the type of dandruff disease you have.

Here are the ingredients for making a dandruff shampoo. First of all, you need to use the base shampoo outlined in chapter 5.

8 oz. plastic clear bottle

Castile liquid soap

MSM torpedoes

Apple cider vinegar

Rosemary herb

Sweet basil herb

Ginger root

Add a tablespoon of each of the following two to three herbs to rosemary and basil and in a jar and mix them well. Once mixed, add three tablespoons of this new mixture to your boiling water.

Here is a list of herbs that you can use for your

dandruff shampoo. Once you make a shampoo and use it up, you should experiment with the other herbs shown here or in the chapter listing all the herbs you can use.

Allantoin

You can also add Allantoin to this dandruff shampoo. Allantoin is a chemical that is naturally produced by many animals, plants, and bacteria. It is used in lotions, skin creams, oral hygiene products, cosmetics, and other toiletries.

Allantoin has no smell, is non-toxic, safe, and non-allergenic. It is a crystalline powder, which softens the skin. This helps the skin to heal quicker and is useful for dry skin and for healing wounds, burns, and scars. **Get Allantoin here.**

After creating your shampoo, also shake it just before using it.

Aloe Vera powder or gel – heals skin burns and promotes cell regeneration and healing.

Aloe Vera gel is an excellent substance to use in your shampoos. Aloe makes your hair thicker, increases its strength and allows your scalp pores to breathe. It adds body and shine to your hair. Put a tablespoon or more of aloe Vera into your shampoo after it has cooled down. You can experiment with different amounts.

Chamomile - contains fatty acids, amino acids, and choline. It has a sedative and emollient effect and normalizes rough skin. It has bacterial and fungicidal properties.

Fennel - has oleic acid and linolenic acid with high levels of tocopherols, flavonoids, protein, sugars vitamins, calcium and potassium. It is an antibacterial and has cytotoxic properties. It is frequently used as a fragrance.

Garlic – provides scalp circulation and promotes hair growth. It also heals scalp irritations, controls flaking and heals eczema.

Lavender - can be used as a fragrance. It controls the production of sebaceous gland oil and reduces itchy and flaky scalp conditions.

Primrose Evening oil - bark and leaves are used for dry hair, dry skin, and eczema.

Rosemary – heals scalp irritations such as eczema and flaking. It also stimulates the scalp. **Use for dark hair, since it may have a darkening effect on light colored hair.**

Thyme – is helpful for itchy and flaking scalps.

Dandruff Shampoo With Oils

You can make a dandruff shampoo by using 8 oz. or 16 oz. of the base shampoo and adding any of the three essential oils.
8 drops of lemon oil
8 drops of rosemary oil
8 drops of rose geranium oil
8 drops of Jojoba oil
8 drops of cade oil
8 to 12 drops of tree tea oil

Shake this shampoo each time you are ready to use it.

Hair Loss Shampoo

When you are experiencing hair loss, you need to shampoo every day with a product that has good natural ingredients. Many people think that shampooing every day, when you have hair loss, harms your hair and accelerates your hair loss. This may be true with commercial shampoos, but not with the shampoos you make.

Many people only rinse their hair with water at the end of their day and think this is ok. You can't just rinse your hair with water at the end of the day to avoid shampooing. When you rinse your hair with water, this allows the sebum trapped in your follicles to increase. This sebum also contains grime and dirt that has collected during the day. This buildup of sebum in your follicles will only worsen your hair loss condition. Daily shampooing is necessary to keep your scalp and hair clean.

To create a hair-loss shampoo, add to the base shampoo any of the following herbs.

Hair Loss

Bearsfoot - is used as treatment for hair loss and usually mixed with jojoba oil or lanolin.

Cinchona bark red or yellow - is used to stimulate growth and reduce oiliness.

Fenugreek - is a good source sapogenins and contains choline, lysine, tryptophan, vitamins A, B and C. It serves as a good source for hair growth tonics.

Ginger - contain lecithin, fatty acids protein, vitamins, and minerals. It is a stimulant for the vascular system and can provide some blood circulation activity in your scalp.

Ginseng - contains many different chemicals that the body needs. It has sterols, pectin, vitamin B12 nicotinic acid, pantothenic acid, biotin, choline minerals like zinc, copper, manganese, calcium, and iron and many more minerals. It can be used in shampoos for hair stimulation and growth.

Licorice – prevents testosterone from converting to DHT in men, which is one of the reasons men lose hair.

Nettles – acts as a blood purifier, blood stimulator, contains a large source of nutrients for hair growth.

7: Herbs To Use In Your Shampoos

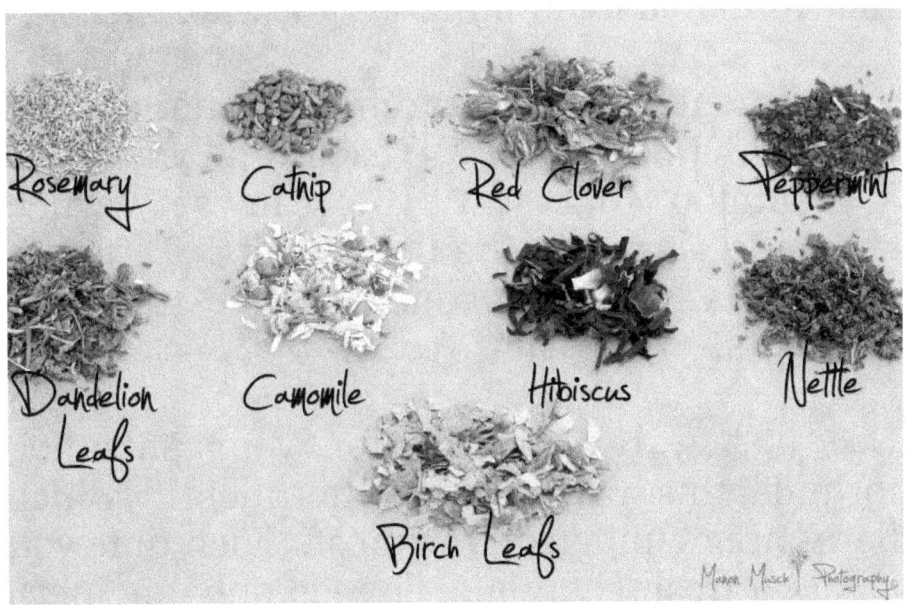

Here is a list of different herbal roots or leaves that you can use in your shampoos. Look for the conditions that you are trying to correct in your hair and choose the appropriate one. If you have sensitive scalp, then you want to add those herbs to your shampoo that have a soothing effect on your scalp, such Aloe Vera or other herbs.

If you want your shampoo to help with hair loss and hair growth, then pick a few of the herbs related to this problem and do a tea infusion. You should also pick those herbs that contain a lot of minerals and vitamins.

Experiment with the different herbs and change the herbs you use each time you make a shampoo that way you can see which shampoo gives you the best results. Different herbs also expose your hair to different nutrients.

Use just 3 to 4 herbs for your shampoo formula, this way you can better identify which herbs are helping you the most. Each time you create a fresh shampoo, change only one herb that way you can tell how your new shampoo is working on your hair. When you find a good combination of herbs that work, use that combination for as long as you want. Herbal shampoos are not like commercial shampoos where you need to rotate from shampoo to shampoo.

Here is the list of great Herbs for scalp and

hair.

Fragrance

Mints such as **peppermint**, **spearmint** are used as fragrances. They are also a scalp stimulant and antiseptic.

Healing Skin

Aloe Vera powder or gel – heals skin burns and promotes cell regeneration and healing. In full strength, Aloe Vera makes hair smoother and manageable. It moisturizes hair and creates a shine.

Hair Tonic and Health

Aritha (Soapnuts) – has proven to be an excellent hair and scalp tonic. It has antifungal and antibacterial properties, so it makes it good for dandruff. It can make your hair feel thicker and silky.

Arnica – contain linolenic acid, vitamins A, B, C, and D. Used as a hair tonic and as a fragrance.

Balsam Tolu – contain cinnamic and benzoic acids. It has a mild antiseptic property and is used for fragrance.

Coltsfoot contains silica and cysteine which is beneficial for hair health.

Hawthorn - is an astringent and can be used as a hair tonic.

Horsetail – contains silica which strengthens your hair shaft. It also stimulates blood circulation of your scalp.

Kelp - contains a high level of mineral salts, vitamins and amino acids that are good for hair health.

Lemon grass - has been used as a fragrance, but also has minerals.

Marshmallow root – provides hair with a conditioning effect.

Oatstraw – is a nutritive herb that has many minerals for your hair. It is useful for hair, boils, skin problems and wounds.

Parsley – promotes your sebaceous gland and hair health.

Anti-Inflammatory

Barberry – is used for an itching scalp, ringworms, and skin disorders.

Comfrey root - contains Allantoin and this chemical has anti-inflammatory, astringent, demulcent and emollient properties.

Elderflower – has anti-inflammatory properties and heals scalp irritations. It is also a soft hair stimulant.

Antiseptic

Golden Seal – has anti-bacterial and antiseptic properties. It can be used for scalp irritations or inflammations, ringworms, psoriasis, skin disorders, ulcers, and wounds.

Oregon Grape – is antiseptic. It helps to heal eczema, psoriasis, and other skin diseases.

Plantain – is anti-inflammatory, and antiseptic. It is good for boils, infections, skin infections or irritations, sores.

Sarsaparilla – is antiseptic. It can be used for eczema, psoriasis, ringworms, skin eruptions, and Hair Growth.

Anti-Bacterial, Anti Pathogenic, Anti – Fungal

Basil – has a high concentration of vitamin A and C and magnesium. The magnesium protects your hair from breakage. It is also as a fragrance. It is also used as an anti-wormal and insect repellent. Basil moisturizes and can add luster to your hair.

Chamomile - contains fatty acids, amino acids, and choline. It has a sedative and emollient effect and normalizes rough skin. It has bacterial and fungicidal properties. It can add highlights to light hair and provides sheen for dark hair. Use it to strengthen the scalp when your scalp has inflammation.

Eucalyptus – has antibiotic, anti-inflammatory, and antiseptic properties. It can be used to treat boils, ulcers, and wounds.

Fennel - has oleic acid, linolenic acid with high levels of tocopherols, flavonoids, protein, sugars vitamins, calcium and potassium. It is has antibacterial and anti-cytotoxic properties and is used as a fragrance.

Juniper – is anti-fungal. It helps when you have boils, fungal infections, hair loss, and worms.

Red Clover – is antibiotic, anti-inflammatory, anti-fungal, and anti-microbial. It can be used for psoriasis, skin disorders, sores and skin wounds.

USNEA – is anti-fungal, anti-bacteria, and antibiotic. It can be used for hair and scalp health, and ringworms.

Hair Loss

Amla – promotes new hair growth and is good for hair loss, since it normalizes blood flow. It is able to penetrate the scalp to strengthen your hair at its root.

Bearsfoot is used as treatment for hair loss

and usually mixed with jojoba oil or lanolin.

Cinchona bark red or yellow - is used to stimulate growth and reduce oiliness.

Fenugreek - is a excellent source sapogenins and contains choline, lysine, tryptophan, vitamins A, B and C. It serves as a good hair growth tonic.

Ginger - contain lecithin, fatty acids protein, vitamins, and minerals. It is a stimulant for the vascular system and can provide some blood circulation in your scalp.

Ginseng - contains many different chemicals that the body needs. It has sterols, pectin, vitamin B12 nicotinic acid, pantothenic acid, biotin, choline. It has minerals like zinc, copper, manganese, calcium, and iron and many more minerals. It can be used in shampoos for hair stimulation and growth.

Licorice – prevents testosterone from converting to DHT in men, which is one of the reasons men lose hair.

Nettles – acts as a blood purifier, blood stimulator, contains a large source of nutrients for hair growth

Sassafras – is used for hair growth and various skin diseases.

Preservative
Apple Cider Vinegar – not a herb but can be used as a shampoo preservative.

Benzoin gum – is used as a preservative and has antioxidants.

Bhringraj (Ecliptaalba) – is an Ayurvedic herb that has been used for centuries for hair loss and premature graying. It helps with skin allergies and is good for rejuvenating hair. This is a great herb to add to your shampoo, since it will strengthen your hair shaft and help with dandruff.

Oily Hair

Betulla – is used for greasy or oily hair. It has anti-inflammatory properties and is also used as a fragrance.

Chickweed – helps to break down oils. It also helps when you have boils, itching, psoriasis, skin diseases, skin rashes, and sores. This herb can also be used in your shampoo for dandruff or for scalp irritating conditions.

Lemon balm – helps to remove excess oil and sebum.
Lemongrass – helps to clean your scalp by removing excess oil and sebum.

Sage – will reduce the formation of sebum in

the sebaceous glands and provides scalp circulation.

Yarrow – reduces the production of sebum in the sebaceous glands.

Scalp

Birch – gives relief for scalp problems such as eczema, boils, and worms.

Burdock Root –it is rich in fatty acids that promote blood circulation to your scalp and it promotes hair growth. It contains silica and phytosterols that soothe irritated scalps. It is good also for dandruff. It can be used to detangle hair and give body to limp hair.

Chaparral – increases the circulation of your scalp.

Comfrey leaves – gives relief to an irritated scalp. It can give life to lifeless hair. It can also be used as a rinse as described in the Hair Rinse Chapter.

Eucalyptus – heals scalp irritation. It can help in regulating sebum production and cleans scalp and pores. It is also an anti-inflammatory.

Figwort – is an anti-inflammatory herb. You can use it to treat eczema, scabies, and rashes.

Hyssop - can be used for treating scalp irritations, burns, or psoriasis.

Nettles or Stinging Nettles – cleans and stimulates the scalp.

Sage - is used as a skin purifier and toner in shampoos. It is for greasy skin and provides fragrance. It has microbial action.

Yarrow - has a soothing effect on the skin and is anti inflammatory and non phototoxic.

Yellow Dock – can be used for itchy skin and various skin eruptions, such as eczema or sores.

Dandruff

Black Walnut Hulls – can be used for dandruff, eczema, skin rashes, pin worms, ringworms, skin diseases, and worms. **DO NOT USE BLACK WALNUT, IF YOU HAVE LIGHT COLORED HAIR.** The hulls are a natural hair dye that darkens hair. This herb will darken your hair. If you have dark hair, then this is not a problem. This herb is also great for oily hair.

Calendula – is anti–inflammatory and antiseptic. It helps the skin when you have bug bites, burns, injuries, skin irritations, skin ulcers, sores, and wounds. It is high in minerals that protect your hair from free radicals and can make your scalp less acidic.

Dandelion Root – is great for dandruff or dry hair. It is an herb rich in minerals, especially iron. It is good sources of vitamin A that will help keep sebum balanced. It can also be used as a hair rinse.

Garlic – provides scalp circulation and promotes hair growth. It also heals scalp irritations, controls flaking and heals eczema.

Lavender - can be used as fragrance. It controls the production of sebaceous gland oil and reduces itchy and flaky scalp conditions

Primrose Evening oil bark and leaves are used for dry hair, dry skin, and eczema.

Rosemary – heals scalp irritations such as eczema and flaking. It also stimulates the scalp. **Use for dark hair, since it may have a darkening effect on hair. If you have light colored hair, use another herb in your base shampoo, like chamomile.**

Thyme – is helpful for itchy, flaking scalps, and has powerful antiseptic properties.

Willow – is antiseptic and anti-inflammatory. It can be used for dandruff, eczema, and wounds.

Yucca – is anti-bacterial and anti-inflammatory and can be used to treat dandruff. It is useful for scalp, skin irritations and inflammations. It has lathering properties, when mixed with water and is frequently used as a soap.

8: Oils And Nutrients To Use In Your Shampoos

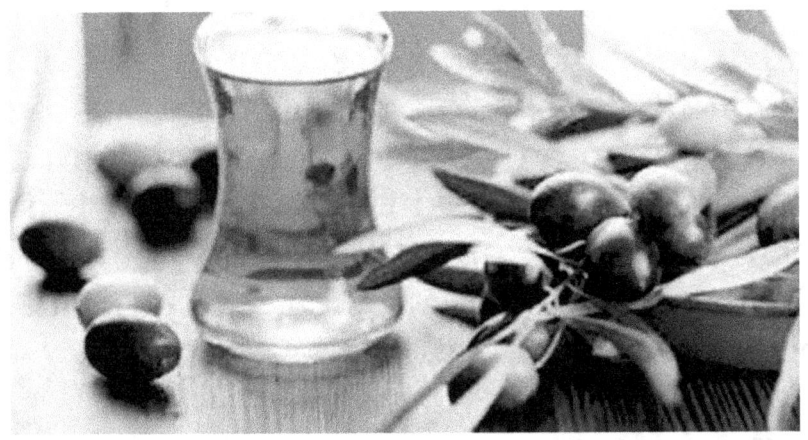

Essential Oils that add fragrance

Here are some herbal essential oils that you can add to your shampoos. You only need to add around 4 to 5 drops of each oil in a 8 oz. bottle of shampoo and around 10 drops in a 16 oz. bottle. You can experiment with the amount you might need, but start out with a small amount then add more after you shampoo, if you feel you need more.

Many of the oils have over lapping properties

just like herbs do. So, go through the list of oil properties and use the ones that you feel will help you.

Many people have some reaction to oils or are allergic to them. You may want to test your reaction to an oil you plan to use, if you know you have sensitive skin. You can do this by placing a small drop of the oil you want to use on your skin. You can then check it in 24 hours for any skin reaction.

Normal Hair

Patchouli
Juniper Berry

Hair Growth
Rosemary
Jojoba

Oily Hair
Lemon
lavender
Bergamot
Juniper

Rosemary
Thyme

Dry Hair
Avocado oil
Carrot seed oil
Jojoba oil
Coconut oil
Olive oil
Tree tea oil

Dandruff Hair

Cade oil
Orange oil
Ginger oil

Avocado oil - contains glycerides of oleic acid amino acids and vitamin D and potassium. Avocado oil is used in many hair products. You can use it for dry hair.

Bergamot oil – is antiseptic and anti-inflammatory and is used for skin afflictions. If you have sensitive skin, you do not want to use this oil. It typically is not used because it is expensive.

Carrot seed oil – is helpful for dry hair.

Cade oil - is effective in shampoos for dandruff treatment. It is also used for eczema, wounds, and parasitic skin. It contains cadinene, cadinol, pcresol, and many other such chemicals.

Coconut and olive oil – protect the hair shafts from water evaporation. They also produce a smooth and shiny hair appearance. You can add a tablespoon of coconut oil into your basic shampoo, if you have dry hair.

Ginger oil - has many benefit for your hair. It is effective for hair loss. It has many vitamins and minerals such as phosphorus and zinc, which treat brittle, dry, or damaged hair. This oil is useful for dandruff when used with olive oil and left overnight on your scalp.

And when ginger, jojoba and avocado oil are mixed and left overnight on your scalp, it helps to increase hair growth rate.

Grapeseed oil - can be used as a preservative and as an antibacterial.

Jojoba oil - is known for helping when you have alopecia or have a scalp condition of various types. Jojoba oil is very similar to sebum and tends to pull out excess sebum from your follicles. Follicles see jojoba oil on the scalp as excess oil and will not produce more. It also reduces scalp irritations and skin flaking. This oil can be a benefit for dry, damaged or brittle hair. This oil can be used for dandruff.

Juniper Berry – is antiseptic and helps to clean your scalp.

Lavender oil - can be used as a fragrance, for hair falling out, and for dry hair.

Lemon oil - can be used as fragrance

Orange oil - is anti-inflammatory, anti-bacterial, anti-fungal and can be used as a fragrance. It contains a variety of mineral, vitamins, oils, and antioxidants that contribute to hair health.

Patchouli – has a dirty, musky smell some people don't like, but when mixed with other oil with good fragrance, it become tolerable or un-noticed. It is used for dry, old, and wrinkled skin and serves as a tissue regenerator. It is antiseptic and anti-inflammatory. Useful for dandruff shampoos.

Rosemary – helps stimulate hair growth. To get an even more powerful oil mixture use jojoba and basil oil with it. Great for dandruff and brittle hair.

Tree tea oil – this oil has antiseptic properties that come from its terpene chemicals. These chemicals penetrate the scalp to provide disinfectant activities at the pore level. Use it for dandruff.

D-Panthenol (Vitamin B5)

D-Panthernol - vitamin B5 helps to

strengthen your hair, grow your hair, and can give your hair a nice shine. This is one of the vitamins that are known to penetrate the hair shaft and be of value in your shampoo.

There is some question about whether vitamins A, D, E, and B can be absorbed by the scalp or hair shaft. For this reason, MSM is added to the base shampoo to serve as a delivery system for the nutrients that are in the herbs. MSM help these vitamins and minerals to penetrate the scalp and hair shaft.

9: Final Natural Hair Rinses

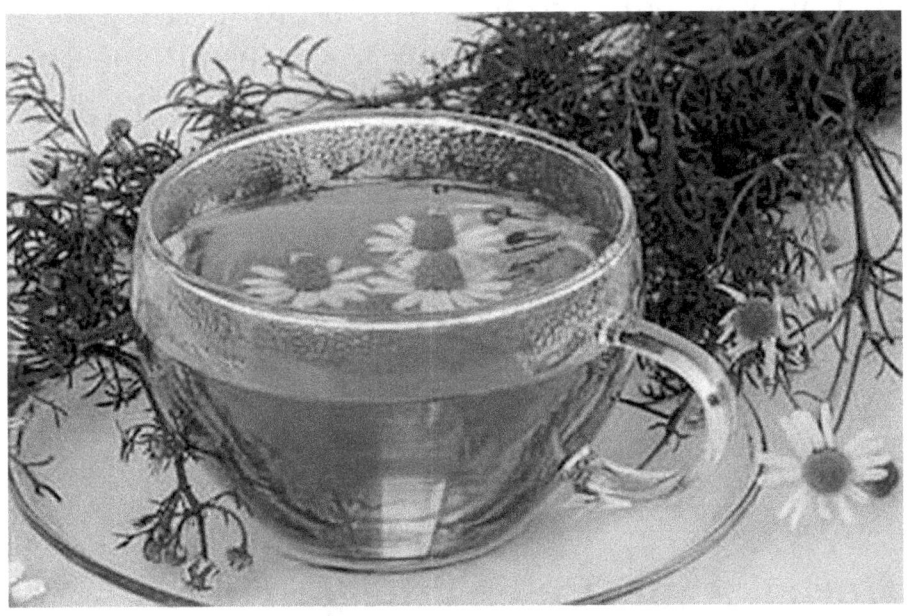

The reason to use a hair rinse after you use a commercial shampoo or conditioner is to remove the shampoo residues that remain on your scalp and hair. When you use the natural shampoos that you have created, residues are not a big problem. But you still want to use a hair rinse, so that you can clean your hair of any residues that might exist and to make your scalp more acidic.

Apple Cider Vinegar Rinse

Mix 50:50 apple cider vinegar with distilled water. You can use less apple cider vinegar, if you feel this is too strong for you. Place this mixture in a plastic bottle and shake to mix. You can use this mixture after you shampoo on your scalp to make your scalp slightly acidic. Let the rinse stay on your scalp for 1 to 2 minutes or so, and then rinse it off with water.

You can store this apple cider rinse in the refrigerator for around two weeks, before you need to prepare another batch.

Herbal Apple Cider Vinegar rinse

Take apple cider vinegar and place it into a pot to make a herbal solution. Pick three herbs from the chapter on herbs. Pick the herbs you want for your hair issues or just use the herbs you already have. Warm the apple cider vinegar slightly using warm heat, and then turn off the hot plate.

Now, place one big heaping tablespoon of each

herb into the warm cider. Mix well and then put this mixture into a closed container, with a small hole on the top so that pressure will not build-up in the container. You can use a mason jar. Now, let this solution sit for 1 ½ to 2 weeks. After this time, strain and pour this solution into a bottle to use in the shower. Keep this solution in the refrigerator and use it over a two period.

Lemon Rinse

Prepare ¼ to 1/2 cup of water with the juice of one lemon. Use this juice as a rinse after you shampoo. Keep it on your hair for about 2 minutes and then rinse it after you have finished showering. Keep it in the regenerator, when you aren't using it and it should keep for a week.

This rinse will keep your hair soft and shiny.

Lemon – Grapefruit Rinse

To create a lemon or grapefruit rinse, squeeze two lemon's juice into 16 to 32 oz. of distilled water. You can use grapefruit instead of lemon or you can try a combination of both.

Use this rinse at the end of your shower.

Herbal Hair Rinses

Just like you make a shampoo, you can make an herbal rinse. But all you have to do is to use the herbal tea or infusion. Boil 3 to 4 cups of water. Then pick any of the herbs listed in the herb chapter. You can pick two to three of the herbs.

Then, steep these herbs under low heat for about 10 minutes and allow cooling for another 10 minutes. Filter this mixture, then add 1/4 cup of apple cider vinegar. Bottle this mixture and start using it.

A recommend herbal pick is to use nettle and rosemary for dark hair and chamomile for blonde, light brown, or gray hair. You can also use calendula, which will add shine to your hair. Clove can be used to bring warm tones to brown hair and improve red and auburn highlights. Cloves also provide you with nice scent.

Apple Cider Vinegar with Essential Oils

Take around two cups apple cider vinegar and pour it into a glass bottle. Add 11 drops of the any one essential oil listed in the essential oil chapter. Let this mixture sit for 24 hours in a dark place.

When you are ready to use it, use one tablespoon or more in a cup of water. You can then use this rinse by pouring it over your head when you have finished shampooing and have finished your shower. It is best to leave this rinse on your head and just pat dry it with a towel.

10: How To Use Your Home Made Shampoos

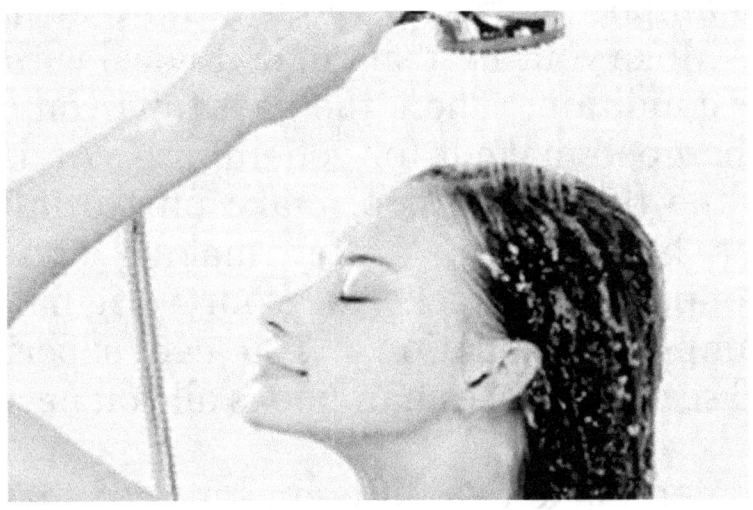

Now, you can make a variety of shampoos. It is best that you vary the types of shampoos you make so that your scalp and hair see a variety of cleansing and stimulating shampoos.

It is always best to use soft water to shampoo your hair. If you have a shower filter that makes your water softer, your hair health will benefit.

Always wet your hair before you shampoo.

Using Shampoos

If you have oily hair it is not good to always use a shampoo that strips your scalp and hair of oil. Make your first shampoo to deal with your oily condition. Then, the next time you create a shampoo make it for general use. And, then for the third shampoo, make one to improve your hair health. After making your 3rd shampoo, go back to your original oily shampoo formulation. You can experiment and see if the base shampoo is all you need.

You can make two different types of shampoo and rotate their use from day to day or from two days to two days.

Different Color Hair

There are certain herbs that you should use if you have dark hair or if you have blond hair. Some herbs that you should use for blond are acacia flowers, black cherry bark, broom, chamomile, marigold flowers, orrisroot, yellow mullein flowers, and quassia chips.

When you make a shampoo, you should test it on a small area of your hair to see if it will change the color of your hair. Herbs that can change the color of your hair are more an issue, if you have light colored hair – blond, red, gray, or light brown. If you have black or dark brown hair, you should not have much of an issue with herbs changing the color of your hair.

Showering With Your Shampoo

When you use the shampoos you made, you will be removing the protective acid layer on your scalp. You will need to restore this layer to protect your scalp. If you use litmus paper to test your shampoo and it tests neutral or slightly acidic, then you scalp will have the right pH.

Massage Hair

When you use your shampoo, pour it onto your hand and not directly onto your scalp. Rub the shampoo into your scalp with gentle, fingertip, massage motion. This will help you eliminate dead skin cells, open up your pores, and stimulate your scalp. Do not use the palms of your hands to massage in your shampoo.

Use your thumbs in an upward, massage motion starting at the lower end of your side burns and up toward the upper side of your hair. This will help to bring blood into the top of your scalp.

Hair massage is necessary, since blood flow to your scalp is typically sluggish and doesn't always provide your scalp and hair with the nutrients it needs.

Oily Hair Shampooing

To make your oily shampoo more effective, create a good lather and leave it on your hair for 3 to 5 minutes. This will give the shampoo time to reduce the oil. If your hair is extra oily, then a second round of shampooing may be necessary.

End Of Shower

You can end your shampooing and showering with a hair rinse. This rinse is to remove contaminates or residues that shampooing leaves in your hair. Most natural shampoos will not leave much residue, but Castile soap may leave some soap residue that you can get rid of with a final hair rinse.

You can use your rinse with a spray bottle to spray the rinse into your scalp. Or, if you have a lot of a hair you may need to have a cup full of rinse to pour over your hair.

After you have showered and have done your final hair rinse, turn off the hot water and end your shower by placing your head in cold water. This will promote blood circulation to your scalp and will provide the basis for better hair health.

But, you can also just use the rinse as your final process and dry your hair slightly to leave the rinse in your hair.

You have a lot of information here on how to create natural shampoos and rinses for your hair. You should experiment with many of these herbs and nutrients to find the best natural shampoo that will keep your hair healthy and scalp free of irritations and dandruff.

Feel free to contact me with your shampoo experiences and this can serve as updates for this book.

11: Resources You Need To Know About

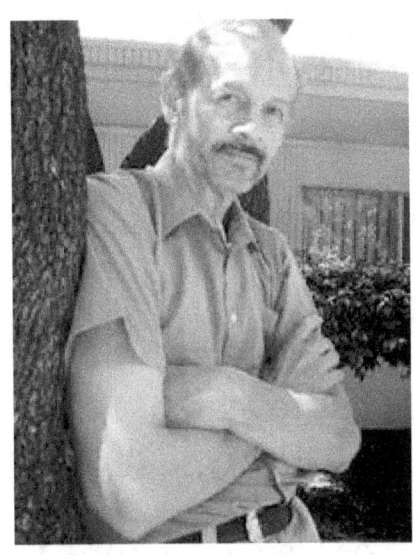

Rudy Silva is a natural consultant nutritionist educated in the United State in Nutrition and Physics. He is a graduate from San Jose State University in California. He is author of 45 other e-books on natural remedies. He has authored a newsletter in natural remedies for over 4 years.

Resource page

Here are some of the other kindle e-books about natural remedies that have been written by this author. You can see the entire list at:

http://tinyurl.com/b2f7wd3

Acne Remedies
Best natural acne treatments: Acne facial

Constipation Remedies
Best Constipated Women Natural Cures
How To Relieve Constipation With Fruits

Essential Fatty Acids
Taking The Mystery Out Of Essential Fatty
acids

Nutrition Remedies
Secret Healthy Fruit Practices Revealed
Fast Healing Juice Nutrition Therapy:
Nutrition Tips 3
Calcium (Discover How To Use Calcium To
Avoid Devastating Diseases)
Magnesium Nutrition Revealed
Best Nutrition Health Practices
Potassium Health Secrets Revealed
A Sodium Diet (What You Must Know About
Sodium)

Stomach Remedies
Acid Reflux: Fast and Easy Cures For Acid
Reflux

Asthma Treatment Cures With Remedies
How To Do Natural Colon Cleansing

Misc Remedies
Natural Hair Loss Treatment: Women And Men
Effective Natural Hemorrhoids Treatment
Iron Deficiency Anemia
Best Impotence Health Diet
What Is A Hiatus Hernia
Best Varicose Vein Treatments?

Men's Health
Best Impotence Health Diet

Weight loss
Ten (10) Day Quick Success Weight Loss Program: A new approach to losing weight by changing your eating habits for life

To see all of the kindle books written by this author, go to this the Authors Profile Page or this URL, http://tinyurl.com/b2f7wd3

If you need support or want to promote any of his e-books, please contact him at rss41@yahoo.com and expect a reply within 24 hours. He looks forward to hearing from you and is happy to help you understand his material on natural and nutritional health.

Give A Review

And, don't for get to give a review for this e-book at Amazon, so that others can gain the benefits of what is in this e-book. A review can be a few sentences.

Rudy S. Silva, Natural Nutritionist

www.ingramcontent.com/pod-product-compliance
Lightning Source LLC
Chambersburg PA
CBHW070756290526
45795CB00002B/576